ENDOMETRIOSIS

THINGS YOU SHOULD KNOW

(QUESTIONS AND ANSWERS)

By Rumi Michael Leigh

Introduction

I would like to thank and congratulate you for purchasing this book, " *Endometriosis, things you should know (questions and answers)*" series.

This book will help you understand, revise and have a good general knowledge and keywords of endometriosis and its effect on the body.

Thanks again for purchasing this book, I hope you enjoy it!

Table of Contents

Introduction..2

Section 1..4

Section 2..6

Section 3..8

Section 4..10

Section 5..12

Section 6..14

Section 7..17

Section 8..19

Section 9..22

Section 10 24

Conclusion 26

Section 1

1) What is endometriosis?

- Endometriosis is the abnormal growth of endometrial tissue outside the uterus.

2) What is the endometrium?

- Endometrium is the lining of the uterus.

3) Can endometrium be found in other parts of the body?

- Yes, endometrium can be found in other parts of the body.

4) What is the main function of the uterus?

- The main function of the uterus is to nourish the fetus.

5) Is there a cure for endometriosis?

- Actually, there is no cure for endometriosis.

6) Is endometriosis contagious?

- No, endometriosis is not contagious.

7) Can endometriosis be prevented?

- No, endometriosis cannot be prevented.

8) Can a woman get pregnant even with endometriosis?

- Yes, a woman can get pregnant even with endometriosis.

9) What part of the body is endometriosis most common?

- Endometriosis is most common on the ovaries.

10) Is endometriosis a chronic disease?

- Yes, endometriosis is a chronic disease.

Section 2

1) What is a chronic illness?

- A chronic illness is an illness that last for a long period of time.

2) Is endometriosis a common health problem?

- Yes, endometriosis is a common health problem.

3) Is endometriosis malign or benign?

- Endometriosis is benign.

4) What is a benign disease?

- A benign disease is a disease that is mild, not harmful, and not cancerous.

5) What is a malign disease?

- A malign disease is a disease that is severe, harmful, and cancerous.

6) Can endometriosis affect women of any age?

- Yes, endometriosis can affect women of any age.

7) What is the origin of endometriosis?

- The origin of endometriosis is unknown.

8) What are some of the hypothesis of the origin of endometriosis?

- Some of the hypothesis of the origin of endometriosis are genetic factors, illness, infection, etc.

9) How many stages of endometriosis are there?

- There are four stages of endometriosis.

10) What are the four stages of endometriosis?

- The four stages of endometriosis are the minimal stage, the mild stage, the moderate stage, and the severe stage.

Section 3

1) What are the risk factors for endometriosis?

- The risk factors for endometriosis include family history, age, menstrual history, an abnormal uterus, etc.

2) Are the symptoms of endometriosis always the same in women?

- No, the symptoms of endometriosis are not always the same in women, symptoms can vary.

3) What are the symptoms of endometriosis?

- The symptoms of endometriosis include period pain, fatigue, pain when urinating during your period, pain when passing stool during your period, pelvic pain, lower back pain, pain during intercourse or after intercourse, constipation, diarrhea, skin issues, depression, mood swings, heavy menstrual periods, nausea, dyschezia, abdominal cramps, anxiety, etc.

4) Is period pain normal?

\- Yes, period pain is normal.

5) What is dysmenorrhea?

\- Dysmenorrhea means painful periods.

6) What is menarche?

\- Menarche is the first menstrual period.

7) What is dyspareunia?

\- Dyspareunia is pain during intercourse.

8) What is dyschezia?

\- Dyschezia is pain experienced during bowel movements.

9) What is the most common symptom of endometriosis?

\- The most common symptom of endometriosis is pain.

Section 4

1) What is ovulation?

- Ovulation is a part of the menstrual cycle. It is the release of mature egg from the ovary.

2) What is the function of the ovaries?

- The function of the ovaries is the production of oocytes and reproductive hormones.

3) What are oocytes?

- Oocytes are eggs.

4) What is ectopic pregnancy?

- Ectopic pregnancy is when a fertilized egg grows outside of the uterus.

5) Ectopic pregnancy can also be called?

- Ectopic pregnancy can also be called extrauterine pregnancy.

6) What is progestogen?

- Progestogen is a steroid hormone that attaches and activates the progesterone receptors.

7) What is estrogen?

- Estrogen is one of the female's sex hormones.

8) What does alcohol do to estrogen levels?

- Alcohol increases estrogen levels.

9) What is progesterone?

- Progesterone is a female steroid hormone released by the ovaries.

Section 5

1) What is amenorrhea?

- Amenorrhea is defined as the absence of menstruation.

2) What is menstruation?

- Menstruation is a normal process of discharge of blood from the tissues of the uterus through the vagina in a woman's monthly cycle.

3) Menstruation is also called?

- Menstruation is also called period.

4) When does menstruation begin?

- Menstruation begins during puberty.

5) When does menstruation end?

- Menstruation ends during menopause.

6) What are the side effects of insufficient estrogen levels for women?

- The side effects of insufficient estrogen levels for women include fatigue, hot flashes, mood swings, osteoporosis, vaginal dryness, etc.

7) What is a hot flash?

- A hot flash is a sudden sensation of intense warmth in the upper part of the body.

8) Can hot flashes be treated?

- Yes, hot flashes can be treated.

9) What is the treatment for hot flashes?

- Hot flashes can be treated with medications or hormone therapy.

10) What is hormone therapy?

- Hormone therapy is a therapy that consists of the utilization of estrogen or/and progesterone.

Section 6

1) What is osteoporosis?

- Osteoporosis is an abnormal loss of bone density.

2) What is an important risk of osteoporosis?

- Osteoporosis can lead to bone fracture.

3) What is menopause?

- Menopause is the natural end of a woman's menstrual cycle.

4) What is urostomy?

- Urostomy is a surgical procedure that creates an opening in the abdominal wall that allows urine to pass through.

5) What is colostomy?

- Colostomy is a surgical procedure that creates an opening called stoma in the colon.

6) What is an endometrial implant?

- An endometrial implant is endometrial tissue that grows outside the uterus.

7) What are viscera?

- Viscera are the internal organs of the body.

8) What is episiotomy?

- Episiotomy is a surgical incision made in the perineum during childbirth.

9) Episiotomy could also be called?

- Episiotomy could also be called perineotomy.

10) What is perineum?

- Perineum is the region between the vagina and the anus.

11) What is fibrosis?

- Fibrosis is the process of scarring of a tissue.

12) What is a scar tissue?

- A scar tissue is the tissue that replaces healthy and damaged tissue. It is a natural healing process of the body.

13) What are uterine fibroids?

- Uterine fibroids are benign tumors located in the uterine wall.

Section 7

1) What are the common complications of endometriosis?

- The common complications of endometriosis include infertility, bladder issues, bowel issues, ovarian cysts, etc.

2) What is an ovarian cyst?

- An ovarian cyst is a pocket or sac filled with fluids in or on the ovary.

3) Are ovarian cysts common?

- Yes, ovarian cysts are common.

4) Ovarian cyst is also known as?

- Ovarian cyst is also known as endometriomas.

5) What is endometrioma?

- Endometrioma is a cyst that is formed when endometrial tissues are found in or on the ovaries.

6) Do ovarian cysts usually require treatment?

- No, most ovarian cysts usually do not require treatment.

7) What are the two main types of ovarian cyst?

- The two main types of ovarian cyst are the functional ovarian cysts and the pathological ovarian cysts.

8) What are functional ovarian cysts?

- Functional ovarian cysts are part of the menstrual cycle and have a short duration.

9) What are pathological ovarian cysts?

- Pathological ovarian cysts are cysts due to abnormal cell growth.

10) What is the most common type of ovarian cysts?

- The most common type of ovarian cysts is the functional ovarian cysts.

Section 8

1) Is there a treatment for endometriosis?

- Yes, there is treatment for endometriosis.

2) What are the treatments for endometriosis?

- The treatments for endometriosis include painkillers, surgery, hysterectomy, hormone medicines, contraceptives, gonadotrophin-releasing hormone (GnRH) analogues, contraceptive implant, etc.

3) Give examples of two common painkillers used for the treatment for endometriosis.

- Paracetamol and ibuprofen are common examples of painkillers used for the treatment for endometriosis.

4) What is the function of gonadotrophin-releasing hormone (GnRH)?

- Gonadotrophin-releasing hormone permits the secretion of follicle-stimulating hormone (FSH) and luteinizing hormone (LH).

5) What are gonadotrophin-releasing hormone analogues?

- Gonadotrophin-releasing hormone analogues are synthetic hormones that decrease the production of estrogen.

6) What is hysterectomy?

- Hysterectomy is the surgical removal of the womb.

7) What is a contraceptive patch?

- A contraceptive patch is a patch put on the skin in order to prevent pregnancy.

8) What is the intrauterine system?

- The intrauterine system is a device that is put in the uterus. This device releases progestogen in order to prevent pregnancy.

9) What is neuropathy?

-   Neuropathy is damage to the nerves.

10) What are neurotransmitters?

-   Neurotransmitters are the chemical messengers of the body.

Section 9

1) What is histology?

- Histology is the study of tissues.

2) How is endometriosis diagnosed?

- Endometriosis can be diagnosed with a CT scan, MRI scan, Ultrasound, and pelvic exams, etc.

3) What is a CT scan?

- A CT scan is a medical imaging that uses computers and rotating X-rays to create images of the body.

4) What is MRI scan?

- MRI scan is a magnetic resonance imaging that creates images of the body using a computer, radio waves and powerful magnetic fields.

5) What is an ultrasound?

- An ultrasound is a medical test that creates an image of the body using sound waves.

6) What is biopsy?

- Biopsy is the removal of tissue sample from the body for medical exams.

7) What is laparoscopy?

- Laparoscopy is a surgical procedure that allows the examination with a camera the interior of the abdomen and pelvis through small incisions.

8) What is cauterization?

- Cauterization is a medical procedure that includes burning a part of the body.

Section 10

1) Do women have testosterone?

- Yes, testosterone can be found in women.

2) What is the function of the fallopian tubes?

- The fallopian tubes connect the ovaries and the uterus.

3) Can scar tissues block the fallopian tubes?

- Yes, scar tissues can block the fallopian tubes.

4) What is the peritoneum?

- The peritoneum is a serous tissue that lines the abdominal walls and covers the abdominal viscera.

5) What are adhesions?

- Adhesions are when organs stick together due to scarring caused by endometriosis.

6) Can endometriosis affect the sciatic nerve?

- Yes, endometriosis can affect the sciatic nerve.

7) What is sciatica?

- Sciatica is pain due to injury to the sciatic nerve.

8) Sciatica is also called?

- Sciatica is also called sciatic neuritis.

9) Sciatic nerve is also called?

- Sciatic nerve is also called ischiadic nerve.

10) What is the longest nerve in the body?

- The sciatic nerve is the longest nerve in the body.

Conclusion

Thank you again for purchasing this book. I hope it has helped you in your journey to understanding endometriosis and its effects on the body.

Please, if you enjoyed this book, I would like you to rate and comment. It'd be appreciated.

Thank you.